THE MODERN MANAGEMENT OF THE MENOPAUSE

A PERSPECTIVE FOR THE 21ST CENTURY

THE INTERNATIONAL CONGRESS, SYMPOSIUM AND SEMINAR SERIES

VOLUME 8

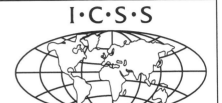

I·C·S·S

ISSN: 0969-2622

THE MODERN MANAGEMENT OF THE MENOPAUSE

A PERSPECTIVE FOR THE 21ST CENTURY

THE PROCEEDINGS
OF THE VII INTERNATIONAL CONGRESS
ON THE MENOPAUSE
STOCKHOLM, SWEDEN 1993

EDITED BY G. BERG AND M. HAMMAR

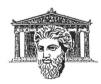

The Parthenon Publishing Group

International Publishers in Medicine, Science & Technology

NEW YORK   LONDON

Published in the UK by
The Parthenon Publishing Group Limited
Casterton Hall, Carnforth,
Lancs, LA6 2LA, England

Published in the USA by
The Parthenon Publishing Group Inc.
One Blue Hill Plaza
PO Box 1564, Pearl River,
New York 10965, USA

Copyright © 1994 Parthenon Publishing Group Ltd

British Library Cataloguing in Publication Data

The Modern Management of the Menopause: A perspective for the 21st Century.—
(International Congress, Symposium & Seminar Series,
ISSN 0969-2622; Vol. 8)
I. Berg, Göran. II. Hammar, Mats. III. Series
612.665
ISBN 1-85070-544-5

Library of Congress Cataloging-in-Publication Data

International Congress on the Menopause (7th : 1993 : Stockholm, Sweden)
 The modern management of the menopause : a perspective for the 21st century /
edited by Göran Berg and Mats Hammar
 p. cm.—(The International congress, symposium, and seminar series, ISSN 0969-
2622; v. 8)
"The proceedings of the VIIth International Congress on the Menopause, Stockholm,
Sweden, June 1993."
Includes bibliographical references and index.
ISBN 1-85070-544-5
 1. Menopause—Congresses. I. Berg, Göran. II. Hammar, Mats. III. Title. IV.
Series.
[DNLM: 1. Menopause—congresses. 2. Estrogen Replacement Therapy—congresses.
WP 580 I61m 1994]
RG186.I57 1993
618.1'75—dc20
DNLM/DLC
for Library of Congress   94-1746
                          CIP

First published 1994

Typeset by Lasertext Ltd., Stretford, Manchester
Printed and bound in Great Britain by
Butler and Tanner Ltd., Frome and London

Contents

Contents

Contents

Contents

Preface

Menopause, the very last menstruation, denotes the end of the reproductive period of life and the beginning of a new era with possibilities to look forward to. Many women pass the climacteric period without any psychological or somatic complaints whereas others suffer from a variety of symptoms.

Peri- and postmenopausal women, i.e. women over 50 years of age, are a rapidly growing proportion of the population and in several countries already constitute 15–20% of the population as a whole. These women carry an increasing responsibility within society, in addition to their traditional family roles.

Approaching the next century, women born in the 1940s constitute those who seek advice for menopausal problems. Today's woman – independent, active and well informed – has the right to be offered the latest information and knowledge to enable her to make an informed decision on her future health.

The menopause and women's health are of rapidly growing concern worldwide. The great scientific interest in this field of healthcare and prevention makes it one of the major health issues of our time. During recent years, some areas within the field of the menopause have generated rapidly growing interest. Such areas are the psychosocial aspects of the menopause, neurobiological phenomena in relation to the changing hormonal situation and cardiovascular effects of hormones, with special emphasis on the direct vascular effects of estrogen. This increasing insight together with the growing epidemiological knowledge on differences between hormone users and non-users makes the field of the menopause an extremely interesting and important area in a general health perspective.

Modern clinical studies illustrate the possibility to adapt treatment regimens to the individual woman and her special demands. Such possibilities include the 'spacing' of progestagen administration, giving continuous combined estrogen/progestagen treatment, using an intra-uterine progestagen delivering device in order to decrease or avoid bleeding, and utilizing alternative administration systems which make hormonal replacement treatment available for new groups of women.

New possibilities to individualize treatment together with professional and empathic information to the woman are probably the most important means to avoid low compliance among women prescribed hormonal substitution treatment.

In June 1993, clinicians and researchers from several different fields gathered in Stockholm, Sweden, for the VIIth International Congress on the Menopause. The most important lectures from invited speakers are summarized in the Proceedings, which thus give a comprehensive overview of the field. The various contributions have been grouped under a number of section headings which to some extent conform with the main symposia of the Congress.

We hope this compilation will be of interest and help for people who are dedicated to research, health and education within the field of the menopause. Increased knowledge within this field will hopefully, in the end, benefit women during a long and potentially active part of their lives, when they can contribute and enrich people and society with knowledge and experience.

Göran Berg   Mats Hammar
Department of Obstetrics and Gynaecology
University Hospital
Faculty of Health Sciences
Linköping
Sweden

List of principal contributors

T. J. Anderson
Department of Pathology
University Medical School
Teviot Place
Edinburgh
EK8 9AG
UK

T. Aso
Department of Obstetrics and
    Gynecology
Tokyo Medical and Dental
    University
School of Medicine
1-5-45 Yushima Bunkyo-ku
Tokyo 118
Japan

A. Ax:son Johnson
The Axel Johnson Group
Box 26008
10041 Stockholm
Sweden

T. Bäckström
Department of Obstetrics and
    Gynaecology
University Hospital
S-90187 Umea
Sweden

G. Berg
Department of Obstetrics and
    Gynaecology
University Hospital
S-581-85 Linköping
Sweden

H. G. Burger
Prince Henry's Institute of
    Medical Research
PO Box 152
Clayton
Victoria 3168
Australia

L. Cardozo
8 Devonshire Place
London
W1C 1PB
UK

C. Christiansen
Centre for Clinical and Basic
    Research
Ballerup byvej 222
DK 2750 Ballerup
Denmark

B. S. Hulka
Department of Epidemiology
School of Public Health
University of North Carolina
CB # 7400, McGavran-
  Greenberg Hall
Chapel Hill
North Carolina 27599-7400
USA

M. S. Hunter
Unit of Psychology
Medical School, Guy's Hospital
London Bridge
London
SE1 9RT
UK

P. A. Kaufert
Department of Community
  Health Sciences
Faculty of Medicine
University of Manitoba
750 Bannatyne Avenue
Winnipeg
Manitoba R3E 0WE
Canada

H. Kuhl
Division of Endocrinology
Department of Obstetrics and
  Gynecology
JW Goethe University
Theodor-Stern-Kai 7
D-6000 Frankfurt am Main
Germany

F. Kuttenn
Department of Endocrinology
  and Reproductive Medicine
Faculte de Medicine Necker
  Enfants Malades
Universite Rene Descartes
Hôpital Necker
149 rue de Sèvres
75015 Paris
France

M. Lachowsky
17 rue Carducci
75019 Paris
France

B.-M. Landgren
Department of Obstetrics and
  Gynaecology
Karolinska Hospital
S-104 01 Stockholm
Sweden

K. A. Matthews
Department of Psychiatry
University of Pittsburgh
3811 O'Hara Street
Pittsburgh
PA 15213
USA

L.-Å. Mattsson
Associate Professor
Department of Obstetrics and
  Gynaecology
East Hospital
University of Göteborg
S-416 85 Göteborg
Sweden

N. L. McCoy
1807 St Louis Drive
Honolulu
HI 96816-1932
USA

B. S. McEwen
Laboratory of
    Neuroendocrinology
The Rockefeller University
1230 York Avenue
New York
NY 10021-6399
USA

M. Metka
I Department of Obstetrics and
    Gynecology
University of Vienna
Spitalgasse 23
A-1090 Vienna
Austria

J. H. J. M. Meuwissen
Department of Gynecologi
St Joseph Hospital
PO Box 7777
5500 MB Veldhoven
The Netherlands

L. E. Nachtigall
251 East 33rd Street
New York
New York 10016
USA

M. Notelovitz
Women's Medical and
    Diagnostic Center and The
    Climacteric Clinic, Inc.
222 S.W. 36th Terrace, Suite C
Gainesville
Florida 32607
USA

J. O'Leary Cobb
President
A Friend Indeed Publications,
    Inc.
3575 Boul. St-Laurant, No. 402
Montreal
Quebec, H2X 2T7
Canada

C. M. Oakley
Clinical Cardiology
Department of Medicine
Hammersmith Hospital
The Royal Postgrad School,
Duncane Road
London
W12 0NN
UK

T. Ohkura
Department of Obstetrics and
    Gynecology
Koshigaya Hospital
Dokkyo University School of
    Medicine
2-1-50 Minami-Koshigaya
Koshigaya
Saitama 343
Japan

A. Oldenhave
Academic Hospital Utrecht
Department of Obstetrics and
  Gynecology
Heidelberglaan 100
3584 CX Utrecht
The Netherlands

I. Persson
Cancer Epidemiology Unit
University Hospital
S-751 85 Uppsala
Sweden

P. M. Sarrel
Department of Obstetrics and
  Gynecology
Division of Mental Hygiene
Box 1505-A
Yale Station
New Haven, Connecticut 06520
USA

W.-B. Schill
Department of Dermatology and
  Andrology
Justus Liebig University
Gaffkystrasse 14
D-35385 Giessen
Germany

J. Sciarra
Department of Obstetrics and
  Gynecology
North Western University,
  Medical School
Room 490
333 East Superior Street, Suite
  490
Chicago, Illinois 60611
USA

B. B. Sherwin
Department of Psychology and
  Obstetrics and Gynecology
McGill University
1205 Dr Penfield Avenue
Montreal
Quebec H3A 1B1
Canada

S. K. Smith
MD MRCOG
Department of Obstetrics and
  Gynaecology
University of Cambridge
Rosie Maternity Hospital
Cambridge
CB2 2SW
UK

S. S. Smith
Department of Anatomy
Institute of Neuroscience
Hahnemann University
Broad and Vine
Philadelphia
PA 19102-1192
USA

G. Tang
Department of Obstetrics and
  Gynaecology
University of Hong Kong
Queen Mary Hospital
Pokfulam Road
Hong Kong

J. A. Tieffenberg
President
Association for Health Research
   and Development
ACINDES
Soler 4829
Buenos Aires (1425)
Argentina

P. Topo
National Research and
   Development Centre for
   Welfare and Health
PO Box 220
SF 00531 Helsinki
Finland

E. Valverius
Experimental Oncology Section
The Radium Home
The Karolinska Institute
S-171 76 Stockholm
Sweden

H. J. J. Verhaar
Research Group for Geriatrics
   and Bone Metabolism
PO Box 85500
3508 GA Utrecht
The Netherlands

A. Vermeulen
Endocrine Department
Medical Clinic
University Hospital
De Pintelaan 185
9000 Gent
Belgium

S. Wasti
Department of Obstetrics and
   Gynaecology
Sultan Qaboos University
   College of Medicine
PO Box 35
Al-Khod Code 123
Muscat
Sultanate of Oman

B. Weiss
1165 Park Avenue
New York
NY 10128
USA

M. Whitehead
Department of Obstetrics and
   Gynaecology
King's College School of
   Medicine
Bessemer Road
London
SE5 9PJ
UK

O. Ylikorkala
Department II Obstetrics and
   Gynecology
University Central Hospital
Haartmaninkatu 2
SF-00290 Helsinki
Finland

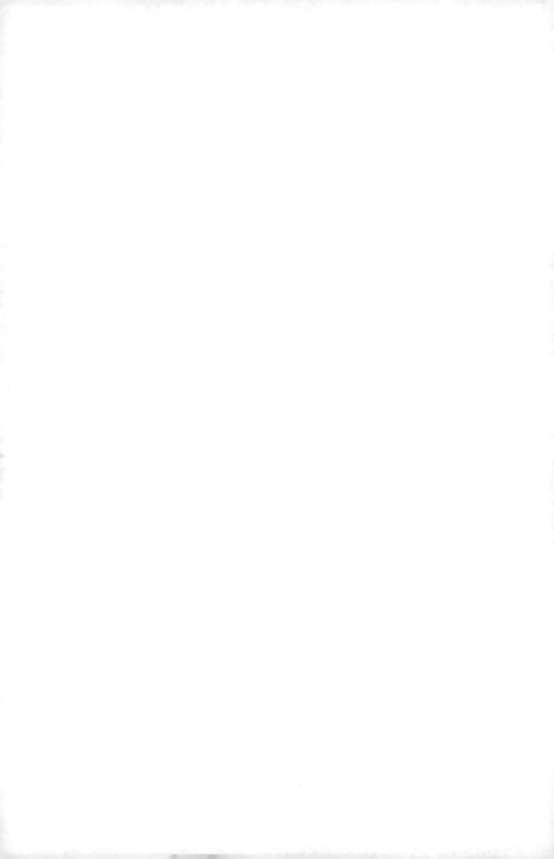

1

The Pieter van Keep Memorial Lecture

INTRODUCTION

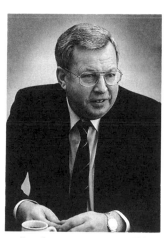 *On 17 June, 1991 Dr Pieter A. van Keep, then President of the International Menopause Society passed away at the age of 58. During his whole professional career, his main interest was the menopause and the study of all aspects of the climacteric in women. Together with Bob Greenblatt, he organized – in 1976 and 1978 – the first and the second International Congresses on the Menopause and following that second meeting, Pieter van Keep, together with some of his dear friends who shared his ideas, founded the International Menopause Society.*

In that same year Pieter van Keep made another important contribution to the advancement of science in the field of the climacteric by launching a new journal, Maturitas. *This was to provide a multidisciplinary approach to the menopause and the climacteric, and he became the founding editor. Since the inception of the Society, almost 15 years ago now, both the knowledge about, and the recognition of the climacteric syndrome, and the role of hormone replacement therapy, have increased tremendously. In addition, life expectancy around the world is rising which means that a rapidly increasing number of women will spend an important part of their lives in the 'Golden Age'. It was Pieter's aim, and it is one of the aims of the Society, that this 'Golden Age' for women becomes a happy, healthy age; not only devoid of short- and medium-term complaints such as hot flushes and*

by this time, had moved its headquarters to Brussels) and returned, as International Medical Director, to Organon.

I would now like to review the five major longitudinal psychosocial studies with you. But before we do that, I'd like to go back to Ede where Laszlo Jaszmann, supported and encouraged by Pieter in the mid 1960s, had started off his cross-sectional studies. The 1967 study from Ede was repeated in 1977 and then repeated again in 1987 by Anna Oldenhave. The data from these three studies spanning the 20-year period appear in *Well-being and Sexuality in the Climacteric.* I will just draw, if I may, two sets of information from it. Up to now in this Memorial Lecture, we have considered women as though they were all intact (i.e. with intact ovaries) but clearly some women will have undergone hysterectomy. The effect of hysterectomy on reporting of symptoms and how it affects them, not only during the climacteric but at other times, must be considered.

Over this 20-year period of investigation, if they had undergone hysterectomy, the Ede data showed that women from their late 30s to early 60s report more moderate and severe flushes.

In terms of severe aches and atypical complaints (a compilation of 21 different symptoms, including restlessness, irritability, etc.) it was found that from the age of 40 through to 60, 'hysterectomized' women do less well than apparently non-hysterectomized women and that their problems predated the hysterectomy. This led Anna Oldenhave to conclude that women who eventually come to surgery have long-standing problems and make more use of medical resources, eventually ending up with a gynecologist who, because he/she has no other alternative, offers a hysterectomy. This really doesn't help because their problems continue thereafter. We will return to this later on.

Now, back to the longitudinal studies. Four of these studies are reviewed by their first authors in the recent edition of *Maturitas*; the principal authors are Holte from Norway, Hunter from England, Kaufert from Manitoba and McKinlay from Massachusetts. The fifth study is by Matthews and colleagues from Pittsburg, Pennysylvania

I can only give you a flavor of these studies. I am briefly going to show what I think are the more interesting data from each of these studies. Beginning with Arne Holte's data – the climacteric was associated with an increase in vasomotor complaints, vaginal dryness, palpitations, and social dysfunction, a reduction in headaches and breast tenderness, and no change in depression, anxiety, and irritability.

Myra Hunter, working in the southeast of London, reported that the climacteric was associated with vasomotor symptoms and sleep problems. And factors which predicted vasomotor symptoms were premenopausal